DIABETES COOKBOOK for NEWLY DIAGNOSED:

Easy and Delicious Recipes to Help you Manage Diabetes

Catherine Megan

INTRODUCTION

Matilda was a young woman who had always been diligent about her health and well-being. She ate nutritious meals, exercised regularly, and took vitamins and supplements to ensure that she was always in top shape. Unfortunately, despite her best efforts, she was diagnosed with Type 2 diabetes.

At first, Matilda was devastated by her diagnosis. She thought her lifestyle choices had failed her and she felt like she had no control over her health any longer. But then she had an epiphany – if she was careful about what she ate and made sure to follow a healthy diet, perhaps she could reverse her diabetes and return to living a healthy lifestyle.

Matilda began researching diets that could help her reverse her diabetes and came across the Mediterranean Diet. She read up on the benefits of this diet and found that it was a well-rounded, balanced way of eating that could help her body heal. She also read about how the Mediterranean Diet is rich in healthy fats, fibers, and essential nutrients which are essential for reversing diabetes.

Armed with this newfound knowledge, Matilda began preparing meals that followed the Mediterranean Diet and began watching her blood sugar closely. To her delight, her blood sugar levels started to drop, and within a few months, she was able to get off all of her diabetes medications and was able to keep her diabetes under control with just diet and exercise alone.

Matilda was amazed by how effective the Mediterranean Diet was in reversing her diabetes and she was so happy to be able to take control of her health. She now follows the Mediterranean Diet every day and encourages others to do the same if they want to reverse their diabetes and enjoy a healthier lifestyle.

Diabetes is a serious, chronic condition that affects the lives of millions of people around the world. It is a disease that affects the human body's ability to produce or use insulin, a hormone that helps the body process and use the sugar found in foods.

Diabetes can cause serious health complications, including heart disease, stroke, kidney failure, and blindness. Despite advances in treatment, diabetes remains one of the leading causes of death in the United States and other countries.

For those living with diabetes, it can be a difficult and challenging condition to manage. But with proper care and support, people with diabetes can lead healthy and fulfilling lives. To begin, it is important to understand the different types of diabetes and the risks associated with each.

Type 1 diabetes, which is often diagnosed in children and young adults, is an autoimmune condition in which the body does not produce enough insulin. Type 2 diabetes, which is more common in adults, is a metabolic disorder in which the body does not properly use the insulin it does produce.

Both types of diabetes can cause serious health complications and require ongoing monitoring and treatment.

It is also important to understand the risks associated with diabetes, such as an increased risk of stroke, heart attack, and kidney disease. A healthy lifestyle with regular physical activity, nutritious meals, and regular medical check-ups can help people with diabetes manage these risks.

Additionally, those with diabetes should monitor their blood sugar levels and take prescribed medications as directed.

Living with diabetes can be difficult, but with the right knowledge, tools, and support, those with diabetes can lead healthy and fulfilling lives. By understanding the different types of diabetes, risks associated with the condition, and how to manage it, those living with diabetes can ensure that they are on the path to a long and healthy life.

Diabetes is a serious and life-altering condition, but with proper management and lifestyle changes, it doesn't have to be a life sentence. One of the best ways to manage diabetes is through cooking.

By understanding which ingredients are best for a diabetic diet, preparing balanced meals at home and experimenting with different flavors, cooking can be an enjoyable way to take control of your diabetes and lead a healthy and active life. So don't be intimidated by diabetes − embrace it, and start cooking!

The goal of this book is to provide an introduction to diabetes, including the different types, risks, and ways to manage the condition. By understanding diabetes and its associated risks, those living with the condition can take steps to manage it and ensure a long and healthy life.

CHAPTER 1

Understanding Your Diabetes

Living with diabetes can be challenging but with proper knowledge and understanding, it can be managed. Diabetes is a condition in which the body does not produce or properly use insulin, a hormone that helps the body use sugar for energy. Without insulin, glucose builds up in the bloodstream, leading to high blood sugar levels.

Diabetes can be managed by understanding the basics of diabetes and how your body works. People with diabetes need to monitor their blood sugar levels regularly, eat a balanced diet, and stay active.

It is also important to know the signs and symptoms of diabetes, such as increased thirst, frequent urination, fatigue, blurred vision, and weight loss. If any of these signs and symptoms are present, it is important to speak with your doctor right away.

Diabetes can also be managed with medication, such as insulin or oral medications. It's critical to comprehend how the medication functions and how to take it correctly. Your doctor will be able to provide you with more information about the medication and how to use it.

Finally, it is important to understand the risks of diabetes, such as heart disease, stroke, and kidney disease. By understanding the risks and how to prevent them, you can make sure that you stay healthy and manage your diabetes.

By understanding the basics of diabetes, you can learn to live with diabetes and manage it successfully.

These tips can help you better understand your diabetes:

• Learn about diabetes and how it affects your body.

• Monitor your blood sugar levels regularly.

• Consume a healthy diet and keep active.

• Be aware of the symptoms and indicators of diabetes.

• Talk to your doctor about medication.

• Understand the risks of diabetes.

• Find support from loved ones and other people with diabetes.

• Make sure to take care of yourself and your diabetes.

Diabetes can be difficult to manage, but it is possible with the right knowledge and understanding.

By taking the time to learn more about your diabetes and how to manage it, you can live a long and healthy life.

Understanding Type 1
What you should know about type 1 diabetes is provided below. Every age, every race, and every shape and size are susceptible to type 1 diabetes. Having it is not shameful, and you have a network of individuals who are willing to assist you.

Working together with your diabetes care team and learning as much as you can about it can provide you with everything you need to flourish.

The body does not manufacture insulin in type 1 diabetes. Your body converts the carbs you consume into blood glucose (also known as blood sugar), which it uses as fuel. Insulin is a hormone required by the body to transport glucose from the bloodstream to the body's cells.

Everyone can learn to manage their disease and live long, healthy lives with the use of insulin therapy and other treatments.

Keep in mind that this illness is treatable. You can live a regular life and accomplish what you set out to do by leading a healthy lifestyle that includes exercise and a balanced diet.

Understanding Type 2

The most prevalent type of diabetes, type 2, occurs when your body improperly uses insulin. Also, while some people may regulate their blood glucose levels with healthy nutrition and exercise, others could require medication or insulin.

Regardless, you have options—and we're here with the tools, resources, and support you need.

A key part of managing type 2 diabetes is maintaining a healthy diet. You need to consume something nutritious that will improve your health while also satisfying your hunger.

Remember, it's a process. Work to find helpful tips and diet plans that best suit your lifestyle—and how you can make your nutritional intake work the hardest for you.

Fitness is another key to managing type 2. The good news is that all you need to do is start moving. The secret is to engage in activities you enjoy as frequently as you can. No matter how physically fit you are, a little exercise each day can help you take control of your life.

Chapter 2

Living with Diabetes

Living with diabetes can be a difficult and complex journey, but with the right support and knowledge, it is possible to live a healthy and active life. Diabetes is a chronic health condition that affects how your body uses the energy from the food you eat. It is caused by a lack of insulin, a hormone that helps the body use glucose (sugar) from the food you eat.

If you have diabetes, it is important to take care of your health by eating a balanced diet, exercising regularly, and monitoring your blood sugar levels. Eating healthy foods and following a meal plan will help you keep your blood sugar levels in a safe range and avoid complications from diabetes.

Exercise is also important for people with diabetes since it can help with weight management and improving overall health.

It is also important to stay on top of your diabetes management. This includes monitoring your blood sugar levels, taking your medications as prescribed, and seeing your healthcare provider regularly. Regularly scheduled appointments with your healthcare provider can help you manage your diabetes and keep it under control.

Living with diabetes can be a challenge, but with the right support and knowledge, it is possible to live a healthy and active life. Make sure to talk to your healthcare provider and get the support you need. Also, remember to take care of yourself and your diabetes. With the right care and management, you can live a long and healthy life with diabetes.

Living with diabetes can be life threatening if not managed properly. It is important to have a regular schedule of blood glucose testing and management, as well as regular physical activity and a balanced diet.

It is also important to have a support system in place to help you manage your diabetes, including family, friends, and healthcare professionals. With the right support and resources, you can learn to manage your diabetes and live a healthy and fulfilling life.

Living with diabetes can be difficult, but it does not have to be overwhelming. With the right attitude and resources, you can lead a full and healthy life.

Chapter 3

Managing Your Blood Sugar

The first step in managing your blood sugar is to understand the basics. Blood sugar is the amount of sugar in your blood, usually measured in milligrams per deciliter (mg/dL).

Between 70 to 100 mg/dL is considered a normal range for fasting blood sugar. If your blood sugar level is higher than this, it is referred to as hyperglycemia.

To help manage your blood sugar, it is important to maintain a healthy diet. Reduce your intake of processed and sugary foods, and focus on eating more whole grains, fruits, vegetables, lean proteins, and healthy fats. It is also essential to get enough physical activity. Exercise helps to reduce blood sugar levels and improve your overall health.

Monitoring your blood sugar levels is also crucial.This can be done by using a blood glucose meter to measure your blood sugar levels. This should be done regularly, especially if you are taking medications to help manage your blood sugar. Keeping track of your blood sugar will help you to identify any issues and make changes to your diet or medication as needed.

Finally, it is important to speak to your doctor about your blood sugar levels and any changes you are making to your diet or medication. Your doctor can provide you with additional tips and advice on how to manage your blood sugar. Together, you can develop a plan that is tailored to your individual needs.

Managing your blood sugar is an important part of maintaining good health. By following a healthy diet, getting enough physical activity, and monitoring your blood sugar, you can help to keep your blood sugar levels in check and prevent long-term health issues.

If you have any questions or concerns, be sure to speak to your doctor.

Chapter 4

Nutrition and Meal Planning

Nutrition is essential for a healthy, balanced lifestyle. Your body gets the vitamins, minerals, and other nutrients it requires to function effectively when you eat a variety of healthy meals.

Furthermore, eating a balanced diet can help maintain a healthy weight, prevent chronic diseases such as diabetes, and reduce the risk of certain types of cancer.

Meal planning is an important part of maintaining a healthy, balanced diet. Planning meals ahead of time helps ensure that you're getting the right mix of nutrients each day. Additionally, meal planning can help save time and money, as it allows you to purchase the necessary ingredients for the week in advance.

When planning meals, it's important to consider portion sizes, the types of foods you're eating, and the number of calories you're consuming.

When planning meals, it's important to focus on nutrient-dense foods such as fruits, vegetables, whole grains, lean proteins, and healthy fats. It's also important to limit or avoid processed foods, sugary beverages, and foods high in saturated fat, salt, and added sugar. Additionally, it's important to stay hydrated by drinking plenty of water throughout the day.

Nutrition and meal planning are essential for maintaining a healthy lifestyle. By focusing on nutrient-dense foods, limiting or avoiding processed foods, and staying hydrated, you can ensure that you're getting the right mix of nutrients each day.

Proteins and lipids do not boost blood sugar as quickly as carbohydrates do. They also have a significant impact on blood sugar levels. The increase in blood sugar following a meal may be reduced by fiber, protein, and fat.

Thus, try to be diverse. Consume a balance of carbohydrates, protein, and fat to better control your blood sugar levels and prolong feeling satisfied. So be cautious to pick nutritious fats and high-quality carbohydrates that are:

- Vegetables, fruits, nuts, beans, peas, and whole grains are high in fiber.
- Seafood such as tuna and salmon are heart-healthy.
- Fruit, vegetables, beans, whole grains, and healthy carbohydrates
- Fish, nuts, seeds, avocado, olives, extra virgin olive oil, and canola oil are examples of healthy fats.

After eating, check your blood sugar. Analyze the relationships between your blood sugar levels and the foods and beverages you consume. Moreover, you might want to keep track of how many servings or grams of carbohydrates you consume with each meal and try to maintain a consistent pattern from meal to meal. You can control your blood sugar by doing this as well.

Saturated fats: Your blood cholesterol rises as a result of saturated fat. It can be found in high-fat dairy products like butter, full-fat cheese, and ice cream as well as coconut oil and chicken skin. High-fat animal proteins like bacon and sausage also include it.

Trans fats: Are liquid oils that solidify; they are also known as hydrogenated or partially hydrogenated oil. components such as stick margarines and shortening, along with processed foods like certain chips, cookies, and fast food French fries, all include trans fats.

In addition to the cholesterol found naturally in your blood, your body also produces cholesterol from the foods you eat. Beware of egg yolks, liver, and other organ meats, as well as high-fat dairy and animal goods.

Sodium: Be mindful of your salt intake as well. It is a component of a healthy diet for diabetics. It has been demonstrated that eating less sodium can both prevent and treat high blood pressure. Choose foods that are low in sodium by reading the labels.

Making a Food Plan for Diabetes: When you have diabetes, eating a healthy, balanced diet doesn't mean you have to give up tasty items. The recipes and sample menu shown below the Meals are a wonderful source of fiber and offer a decent ratio of protein to fat. Together with the other fruits, vegetables, grains, dairy, proteins, and fats in your diet plan, you can include them in moderation.

Chapter 5

Shopping for Healthy Foods

Focusing on nutrient-dense, low-glycemic foods is vital when choosing a healthful diet for a diabetic patient. This entails staying away from refined carbohydrates, processed foods, and sweet snacks.

Make whole grains, legumes, fruits, vegetables, lean meats, and healthy fats your top priorities instead. Fiber and vital vitamins and minerals are provided by whole grains including quinoa, oats, and brown rice. Additionally a fantastic source of fiber, protein, and complex carbohydrates are legumes like beans and lentils.

Because of their high fiber and vitamin and mineral content, fruits and vegetables are essential for health. Essential amino acids and little saturated fat are provided by lean proteins including fish, chicken, and eggs.

It's critical to balance saturated and trans fats in the diet with healthy fats from foods like nuts, seeds, and avocados.

When shopping, carefully read the labels and look for items with entire ingredients rather than processed ones. Anything with more sugar, sodium, or harmful fats should be avoided. Create a list before you go shopping to help you concentrate on the things you really need and prevent impulse buys.

Look for pre-cut fruits and vegetables, lean proteins that have already been cooked, and whole grain products like quinoa salads and brown rice when shopping for convenience foods.

Eating healthy food is an important part of managing diabetes. Shopping for the right foods can help you create meals that are nutritious, delicious, and supportive of your overall health.

Shopping for healthy foods as a diabetic can feel overwhelming. However, it is important to plan ahead and make smart, informed decisions. Here are some tips to help you get the most out of your shopping trips:

1. Make a list: Before you head to the store, create a list of healthy foods that make up the core of your diet as a diabetic. This should include lean proteins, whole grains, fiber-rich fruits and vegetables, healthy fats, and low-fat dairy.

2. Read labels: Look for foods that are low in sugar and saturated fat, and that have a moderate amount of sodium.

3. *Choose whole grains:* Whole grains are an important part of a diabetic diet, as they provide essential vitamins, minerals, and fiber. Look for items such as brown rice, quinoa, oats, and barley.

4. *Stock up on fresh produce:* Fresh fruits and vegetables are packed with vitamins, minerals, and fiber, and are essential for any healthy diet. Try to buy a variety of produce, such as apples, oranges, broccoli, spinach, and kale.

5. *Avoid processed foods:* Avoid pre-packaged and processed foods, as they are often high in sugar, sodium.

Chapter 6

Recipes

Breakfast

1. Oats and Flaxseed Porridge – 10 minutes
Ingredients:
- ¼ cup oats
- 1 tablespoon of flaxseeds
- 1 cup of skimmed milk
- 1 teaspoon of honey
- 1 tablespoon of dried cranberries
- 2 tablespoons of blueberries

Instructions:
1. In a saucepan, add the oats, flaxseeds and milk, and bring to a simmer over medium heat.
2. Cook for about five minutes, stirring occasionally, until the oats and flax seeds are cooked.
3. Stir in the honey, cranberries and blueberries, and cook for another minute or two until everything is combined and heated through.
4. Serve warm and enjoy!

2. Egg and Spinach Scramble – 10 minutes
Ingredients:
- 2 eggs
- 1 cup of baby spinach
- 1 teaspoon of olive oil

- 1 tablespoon of grated cheese
- Salt and pepper to taste

Instructions:
1. Heat the olive oil in a non-stick frying pan over medium heat.
2. Whisk the eggs in a small bowl and season with salt and pepper.
3. Add the eggs to the pan and cook until they start to set.
4. Add the spinach and cook for another two minutes until the eggs are cooked through.
5. Sprinkle it with cheese and serve.

3. Greek Yogurt with Fresh Fruit – 5 minutes
Ingredients:
- ½ cup of Greek yogurt
- 1 tablespoon of honey
- 1 cup of fresh berries
- 2 tablespoons of chopped nuts

Instructions:
1. Place the Greek yogurt in a bowl and drizzle with the honey.
2. Top with the fresh berries and chopped nuts.
3. Mix everything together and enjoy!

4. Omelette with Mushrooms and Tomatoes – 10 minutes
Ingredients:
- 2 eggs
- 1 tablespoon of olive oil

- 1 cup of sliced mushrooms
- 1 cup of cherry tomatoes, halved
- Salt and pepper to taste

Instructions:
1. Heat the olive oil in a non-stick frying pan over medium heat.
2. Beat the eggs in a small bowl and season with salt and pepper.
3. Add the eggs to the pan and cook until they start to set.
4. Add the mushrooms and tomatoes and cook for another two minutes until the eggs are cooked through.
5. Serve and enjoy!

5. Avocado Toast – 5 minutes
Ingredients:
- 2 slices of whole-wheat bread
- 1 ripe avocado
- 1 teaspoon of olive oil
- Salt and pepper to taste

Instructions:
1. Toast the bread in a toaster.
2. Cut the avocado in half and remove the pit.
3. Scoop the avocado flesh onto the toast and mash with a fork.
4. Drizzle with the olive oil and season with salt and pepper.
5. Serve and enjoy!

6. Low-Fat Banana Pancakes – 10 minutes
Ingredients:
- ¾ cup of whole wheat flour
- 2 tablespoons of sugar
- 1 teaspoon of baking powder
- 1 cup of skimmed milk
- 1 ripe banana, mashed
- 2 tablespoons of olive oil

Instructions:
1. In a large bowl, combine the flour, sugar and baking powder.
2. Add the milk and mashed banana and mix until everything is combined.
3. Heat the olive oil in a non-stick frying pan over medium heat.
4. Drop the batter by the tablespoonful into the pan and cook for about two minutes until golden brown.
5. Flip the pancakes and cook for another two minutes.
6. Serve with honey or your favorite syrup.

7. Vegetable Frittata – 10 minutes
Ingredients:
- 2 eggs
- 1 teaspoon of olive oil
- 1 cup of diced vegetables (e.g. bell peppers, mushrooms, onions, etc.)
- Salt and pepper to taste

Instructions:
1. Preheat the oven to 350°F.

2. Heat the olive oil in a non-stick oven-proof frying pan over medium heat.
3. Add the vegetables and cook for about five minutes until softened.
4. Whisk the eggs in a small bowl and season with salt and pepper.
5. Pour the eggs over the vegetables and cook for two minutes until the eggs start to set.
6. Place the pan in the oven and bake for about five minutes until the eggs are cooked through.
7. Serve and enjoy!

8. Berry and Almond Smoothie – 5 minutes
Ingredients:
- ½ cup of skimmed milk
- ½ cup of plain Greek yogurt
- ½ cup of frozen berries
- 2 tablespoons of chopped almonds
- 1 teaspoon of honey

Instructions:
1. Place all the ingredients in a blender and blend until smooth.
2. Serve and enjoy!

9. Whole-Wheat Toast with Peanut Butter – 5 minutes
Ingredients:
- 2 slices of whole-wheat bread
- 2 tablespoons of peanut butter

Instructions:

1. Toast the bread in a toaster.
2. Spread the peanut butter on the toast.
3. Serve and enjoy!

10. Chia Seed Pudding – 10 minutes
Ingredients:
- ½ cup of chia seeds
- 1 cup of skimmed milk
- 1 teaspoon of honey
- 2 tablespoons of dried cranberries

Instructions:
1. In a bowl, combine the chia seeds, milk and honey.
2. Stir well and let it sit for five minutes until the chia seeds start to absorb the liquid.
3. Stir in the dried cranberries.
4. Cover and refrigerate for at least two hours.
5. Serve chilled and enjoy!

Lunch

1. Avocado and Hummus Wrap: 10 minutes
Ingredients:
- 2 whole wheat tortillas
- 2 tablespoons of hummus
- 1/4 of an avocado, sliced
- 1/4 cup of spinach
- 1/4 cup of diced cucumber
Instructions:

1. Spread the hummus on the tortillas.
2. Top with avocado, spinach, and cucumber.
3. Roll up the tortillas and slice in half.
4. Serve.

2. Baked Salmon with Zucchini: 15 minutes
Ingredients:
- 2 salmon fillets
- 1 teaspoon of olive oil
- 1/2 teaspoon of garlic powder
- 1/2 teaspoon of paprika
- 1/4 teaspoon of ground black pepper
- 1/4 teaspoon of salt
- 2 zucchini, sliced
Instructions:
1. Preheat the oven to 375°F.
2. Place the salmon fillets in a baking dish.
3. Drizzle with olive oil, garlic powder, paprika, pepper, and salt.
4. Arrange the zucchini slices around the salmon.
5. Bake for 10-15 minutes, or until the salmon is cooked through and the zucchini is tender.
6. Serve.

3. Quinoa Tomato Salad: 10 minutes
Ingredients:
- 1 cup of cooked quinoa
- 1/2 cup of diced tomatoes
- 2 tablespoons of diced red onion
- 1 tablespoon of olive oil
- 1 tablespoon of fresh lemon juice
- Salt and pepper, to taste

Instructions:
1. In a large bowl, combine the quinoa, tomatoes, and red onion.
2. Drizzle with olive oil and lemon juice.
3. Season with salt and pepper, to taste.
4. Toss to combine.
5. Serve.

4. Greek Yogurt Parfait: 5 minutes
Ingredients:
- 1 cup of Greek yogurt
- 1/2 cup of granola
- 1/2 cup of fresh berries
Instructions:
1. In a bowl or glass, layer the yogurt, granola, and berries.
2. Repeat with remaining ingredients.
3. Serve.

5. Tuna Salad: 10 minutes
Ingredients:
- 2 (5-ounce) cans of tuna, drained
- 1/4 cup of diced red onion
- 1/4 cup of diced celery
- 2 tablespoons of Greek yogurt
- 2 tablespoons of mayonnaise
- 1 tablespoon of lemon juice
- Salt and pepper, to taste
Instructions:
1. In a large bowl, combine the tuna, red onion, and celery.

2. Add the Greek yogurt, mayonnaise, and lemon juice.
3. Season with salt and pepper, to taste.
4. Toss to combine.
5. Serve.

6. Lentil and Veggie Soup: 15 minutes
Ingredients:
- 1 tablespoon of olive oil
- 1/2 cup of diced onion
- 1 cup of diced carrots
- 1 cup of diced celery
- 2 cloves of garlic, minced
- 1 (14-ounce) can of lentils, drained
- 4 cups of vegetable broth
- 1 teaspoon of dried oregano
- 1/2 teaspoon of dried thyme
- Salt and pepper, to taste
Instructions:
1. Heat the olive oil in a large pot over medium heat.
2. Add the onion, carrots, and celery. Cook for 5 minutes, stirring occasionally.
3. Stir in the garlic and cook for 1 minute.
4. Add the lentils, vegetable broth, oregano, and thyme.
5. Bring the soup to a simmer and cook for 10 minutes, or until the vegetables are tender.
6. Season with salt and pepper, to taste.
7. Serve.

7. Egg and Avocado Toast: 5 minutes

Ingredients:
- 2 slices of whole wheat bread, toasted
- 1/4 of an avocado, mashed
- 2 eggs, cooked to desired doneness
- Salt and pepper, to taste

Instructions:
1. Spread the mashed avocado on the toasted bread.
2. Top with the eggs.
3. Sprinkle it with salt and pepper, to taste.
4. Serve.

8. Quinoa Bowl: 10 minutes
Ingredients:
- 1 cup of cooked quinoa
- 1/2 cup of black beans, cooked
- 1/2 cup of diced bell peppers
- 1/4 cup of diced red onion
- 2 tablespoons of cilantro, chopped
- 2 tablespoons of olive oil
- 2 tablespoons of lime juice

Instructions:
1. In a large bowl, combine the quinoa, black beans, bell peppers, red onion, and cilantro.
2. Drizzle with olive oil and lime juice.
3. Toss to combine.
4. Serve.

9. Shrimp and Asparagus Stir Fry: 10 minutes
Ingredients:
- 1 tablespoon of olive oil
- 1 pound of shrimp, peeled and deveined

- 1/2 teaspoon of garlic powder
- 1/2 teaspoon of paprika
- 1/4 teaspoon of ground black pepper
- 1/4 teaspoon of salt
- 1 bunch of asparagus, trimmed and cut into 1-inch pieces
- 1/4 cup of low-sodium soy sauce

Instructions:

1. Heat the olive oil in a large skillet over medium heat.
2. Add the shrimp and season with garlic powder, paprika, pepper, and salt.
3. Cook for 3 minutes, or until the shrimp is cooked through.
4. Add the asparagus and soy sauce.
5. Cook for another 3 minutes, or until the asparagus is tender.
6. Serve.

10. Broccoli and Cheese Omelette: 10 minutes

Ingredients:

- 2 eggs
- 2 tablespoons of milk
- 1/2 cup of broccoli, cooked
- 1/4 cup of shredded cheddar cheese
- Salt and pepper, to taste

Instructions:

1. In a bowl, whisk together the eggs and milk.
2. Heat a non-stick skillet over medium heat and pour in the egg mixture.
3. Cook for 2-3 minutes, or until the eggs are set.

4. Flip the omelette and top with the broccoli and cheese.
5. Cook for another 2-3 minutes, or until the cheese is melted and the omelette is cooked through.
6. Season with salt and pepper, to taste.
7. Serve.

Dinner

1. Baked Salmon with Asparagus – Prep Time: 10 minutes, Cook Time: 15 minutes
Ingredients:
•4 (4-ounce) salmon fillets
•1 teaspoon extra-virgin olive oil
•1 teaspoon freshly ground black pepper
•1/2 teaspoon garlic powder
•1/2 teaspoon onion powder
•1/2 teaspoon dried basil
•1/2 teaspoon dried oregano
•1/4 teaspoon sea salt
•1 pound asparagus, trimmed
Instructions:
1. Preheat oven to 400°F.
2. Place salmon fillets on a parchment-lined baking pan.
3. Drizzle with olive oil and sprinkle with black pepper, garlic powder, onion powder, basil, oregano, and sea salt.

4. Bake for 12 to 15 minutes, or until the salmon is cooked through.

5. Meanwhile, steam the asparagus until tender, about 8 minutes.

6. Serve the salmon with the asparagus. Enjoy!

2. Grilled Pork Chops with Brussels Sprouts – Prep Time: 10 minutes, Cook Time: 25 minutes

Ingredients:

•4 (4-ounce) boneless pork chops

•1 tablespoon olive oil

•1 teaspoon garlic powder

•1 teaspoon onion powder

•1 teaspoon dried oregano

•1/2 teaspoon dried thyme

•1/2 teaspoon freshly ground black pepper

•1/4 teaspoon sea salt

•1 pound Brussels sprouts, trimmed and halved

Instructions:

1. Preheat a grill to medium-high heat.

2. Brush the pork chops with the olive oil and season with garlic powder, onion powder, oregano, thyme, black pepper, and sea salt.

3. Grill the pork chops for 4 to 5 minutes per side, or until the pork is cooked through.

4. Meanwhile, steam the Brussels sprouts until tender, about 10 minutes.

5. Serve the pork chops with the Brussels sprouts. Enjoy!

3. Veggie Stir-Fry – Prep Time: 10 minutes, Cook Time: 15 minutes

Ingredients:
•1 tablespoon sesame oil
•1 teaspoon garlic, minced
•1 teaspoon ginger, minced
•1 red bell pepper, sliced
•1 green bell pepper, sliced
•1 cup broccoli florets
•1 cup snow peas
•1/4 cup low-sodium soy sauce
•2 tablespoons white vinegar
Instructions:
1. Heat the sesame oil in a large skillet over medium-high heat.
2. Add the garlic and ginger and sauté for 1 minute.
3. Add the bell peppers and sauté for 2 minutes.
4. Add the broccoli and snow peas and sauté for 3 minutes.
5. Add the soy sauce and vinegar and stir to combine.
6. Cook for 2 minutes, or until the vegetables are tender.
7. Serve and enjoy!

4. Quinoa Bowl with Avocado and Black Beans – Prep Time: 10 minutes, Cook Time: 15 minutes
Ingredients:
•1 cup quinoa
•2 cups water
•1 teaspoon extra-virgin olive oil
•1/4 teaspoon sea salt
•1 (15-ounce) can black beans, drained and rinsed
•1 avocado, diced

•1/4 cup chopped cilantro
•1 lime, juiced
Instructions:
1. In a medium saucepan, combine the quinoa and water. Bring to a boil, reduce heat to low, cover, and simmer for 15 minutes, or until the quinoa is cooked.
2. Remove from heat and fluff with a fork.
3. Add the olive oil and sea salt and stir to combine.
4. In a bowl, combine the quinoa, black beans, avocado, cilantro, and lime juice.
5. Serve and enjoy!

5. Baked Cod with Roasted Potatoes – Prep Time: 10 minutes, Cook Time: 30 minutes
Ingredients:
•4 (4-ounce) cod fillets
•1 teaspoon extra-virgin olive oil
•1 teaspoon garlic powder
•1 teaspoon onion powder
•1 teaspoon dried oregano
•1/2 teaspoon dried thyme
•1/2 teaspoon freshly ground black pepper
•1/4 teaspoon sea salt
•2 cups Yukon gold potatoes, diced
Instructions:
1. Preheat oven to 400°F.
2. Place cod fillets on a parchment-lined baking pan.
3. Drizzle with olive oil and sprinkle with garlic powder, onion powder, oregano, thyme, black pepper, and sea salt.

4. Bake for 15 minutes.

5. Meanwhile, toss the potatoes with the remaining olive oil, garlic powder, onion powder, oregano, thyme, black pepper, and sea salt.

6. Place on a parchment-lined baking sheet and bake for 15 minutes, or until the potatoes are golden and tender.

7. Serve the cod with the roasted potatoes. Enjoy!

Snacks and Desserts

1. Apple Pie Bites:
Prep Time: 10 minutes
Ingredients:
- 2 apples, peeled and cubed
- 2 tablespoons of sugar-free maple syrup
- 2 tablespoons of cinnamon
- 2 tablespoons of butter
- 3 tablespoons of almond flour
- 1 teaspoon of vanilla extract
Instructions:
1. Preheat oven to 350°F.
2. Grease a baking sheet with butter.
3. In a medium bowl, mix together the cubed apples, sugar-free maple syrup, cinnamon, butter, almond flour, and vanilla extract.
4. Place the mixture on the baking sheet and spread into an even layer.

5. Bake for 10 minutes until the apple pieces are soft and lightly browned.
6. Allow to cool before serving.

2. Chocolate Peanut Butter Protein Bars:
Prep Time: 10 minutes
Ingredients:
- 2 cups of rolled oats
- 2 scoops of sugar-free protein powder
- 2 tablespoons of cocoa powder
- 1/4 cup of peanut butter
- 1/4 cup of honey
- 1/4 cup of almond milk
- 1 teaspoon of vanilla extract
Instructions:

1. Preheat oven to 350°F.
2. Grease an 8"x8" baking pan with butter.
3. In a medium bowl, mix together the rolled oats, protein powder, cocoa powder, peanut butter, honey, almond milk, and vanilla extract.
4. Pour the mixture into the baking pan and spread into an even layer.
5. Bake for 40 minutes until the bars are lightly browned and set.
6. Allow to cool before cutting into bars and serving.

3. Oatmeal Raisin Cookies:
Prep Time: 10 minutes
Ingredients:
- 1 cup of old-fashioned oats

- 1/4 cup of almond flour
- 1/4 cup of coconut oil
- 1/4 cup of honey
- 1 teaspoon of vanilla extract
- 1/2 teaspoon of cinnamon
- 1/4 cup of raisins

Instructions:
1. Preheat oven to 350°F.
2. Grease a baking sheet with butter.
3. In a medium bowl, mix together the oats, almond flour, coconut oil, honey, vanilla extract, and cinnamon.
4. Fold in the raisins.
5. Place the mixture on the baking sheet and form into 12 cookies.
6. Bake for 10 minutes until the cookies are lightly browned.
7. Allow to cool before serving.

4. Banana Yogurt Parfaits:
Prep Time: 5 minutes
Ingredients:
- 2 cups of plain Greek yogurt
- 2 tablespoons of honey
- 2 bananas, sliced
- 1/2 cup of almonds, chopped

Instructions:
1. In a medium bowl, mix together the yogurt and honey.
2. Layer the yogurt, banana slices, and chopped almonds in two serving cups.
3. Serve immediately.

5. Baked Apple Chips:
Prep Time: 5 minutes
Ingredients:
- 2 apples, cored and thinly sliced
- 1 teaspoon of cinnamon
Instructions:
1. Preheat oven to 250°F.
2. Grease a baking sheet with butter.
3. Arrange the apple slices on the baking sheet and sprinkle with cinnamon.
4. Bake for 30 minutes until the slices are crisp and lightly browned.
5. Allow to cool before serving.

6. Cinnamon Almond Butter Bites:
Prep Time: 5 minutes
Ingredients:
- 1/4 cup of almond butter
- 2 tablespoons of sugar-free maple syrup
- 1 teaspoon of cinnamon
- 1/4 cup of almonds, chopped
Instructions:
1. In a medium bowl, mix together the almond butter, sugar-free maple syrup, and cinnamon.
2. Add the chopped almonds and mix until combined.
3. Form the mixture into 12 balls.
4. Serve immediately.

7. Chocolate Avocado Truffles:
Prep Time: 10 minutes

Ingredients:
- 1 ripe avocado
- 2 tablespoons of cocoa powder
- 2 tablespoons of honey
- 2 tablespoons of almond milk
Instructions:
1. In a food processor, blend together the avocado, cocoa powder, honey, and almond milk until smooth.
2. Form the mixture into 12 truffles.
3. Serve immediately.

8. Yogurt Fruit Popsicles:
Prep Time: 10 minutes
Ingredients:
- 2 cups of plain Greek yogurt
- 2 tablespoons of honey
- 1/2 cup of strawberries, chopped
- 1/2 cup of blueberries
Instructions:
1. In a medium bowl, mix together the yogurt and honey.
2. Divide the mixture evenly into 8 popsicle molds.
3. Top each popsicle with the chopped strawberries and blueberries.
4. Freeze for at least 4 hours until solid.
5. Serve immediately.

9. No-Bake Coconut Energy Balls:
Prep Time: 10 minutes
Ingredients:
- 1/2 cup of unsweetened coconut flakes

- 1/4 cup of almond butter
- 2 tablespoons of honey
- 1/4 cup of almond flour

Instructions:

1. In a medium bowl, mix together the coconut flakes, almond butter, honey, and almond flour.
2. Form the mixture into 16 balls.
3. Place the balls in an airtight container and freeze for at least 2 hours.
4. Serve immediately.

10. Coconut Almond Butter Balls:

Prep Time: 10 minutes

Ingredients:

- 1/2 cup of unsweetened coconut flakes
- 1/4 cup of almond butter
- 2 tablespoons of honey
- 1/4 cup of almonds, chopped

Instructions:

1. In a medium bowl, mix together the coconut flakes, almond butter, honey, and chopped almonds.
2. Form the mixture into 16 balls.
3. Serve immediately.

Chapter 7

Meal Planning Resources

Meal planning is an essential part of a healthy lifestyle. It can help you save time, money, and make sure you're eating nutritious meals. With so many resources available, it's easy to get overwhelmed.

To help you get started, here's a look at some of the best meal planning resources out there.

1. Meal Planning Apps: Meal planning apps are a great way to get organized and plan meals. Some apps even offer meal ideas and recipes, while others provide grocery lists so you know exactly what you need to buy. For example, Mealime and Prepear offer great meal planning solutions.

2. Grocery Delivery Services: If you're short on time, grocery delivery services can be a lifesaver. Many grocery stores offer delivery, or you can use services like Instacart or AmazonFresh to get your groceries delivered straight to your door.

3. Meal Delivery Services: Meal delivery services make meal planning even easier. They provide pre-made meals and ingredients so you can whip up healthy meals in no time. Companies like Blue

Apron and HelloFresh are popular meal delivery services.

4. Cookbooks: Cookbooks are filled with delicious recipes and meal ideas. If you're looking for inspiration, a cookbook is a great resource. Popular cookbooks include The Fit Foodie Meal Plan and Eat Clean, Stay Lean.

5. Meal Planning Websites: Meal planning websites are great for finding recipes, meal ideas, and grocery lists. Popular websites include: MyFitnessPal and All Recipes.

Meal planning doesn't have to be hard. With the right resources, you can easily plan healthy meals that fit your budget and lifestyle. Whether you use meal planning apps, delivery services, cookbooks, or meal planning websites, you'll be sure to find something that works for you.

Chapter 8

Diabetes Support Groups

Diabetes is a serious and often life-threatening condition that requires ongoing management to help people stay healthy. Diabetes support groups are a great way for people with diabetes to connect with each other and share tips, advice, and support.

The primary goal of a diabetes support group is to provide a safe and supportive environment for people with diabetes to discuss their experiences and challenges in managing the condition.

In a support group, members can ask questions, share their own experiences, and receive emotional support from their peers.

Support groups can offer a range of activities and services to help people with diabetes. Many support groups provide educational programs to help members learn about diabetes and its management.

These programs can provide valuable information about nutrition, medication management, and how to best manage blood sugar levels. Additionally, many diabetes support groups offer counseling and support services to help people cope with the emotional challenges of living with diabetes.

It is important to find a support group that is right for you. Different groups may offer different activities and services, so it is important to research the different options and find one that best meets your needs.

It is also important to find a group that is active and welcoming so that you can benefit from the experience of other members.

In addition to attending a diabetes support group, there are other ways to connect with people who have diabetes. There are many online support groups that offer information and support for people with diabetes.

Additionally, there are many resources available to help people with diabetes find support and information, such as websites, forums, and blogs.

Living with diabetes can be difficult, but having access to a supportive community can make a huge difference. Diabetes support groups provide an important resource to help people manage the condition and improve their quality of life.

Support groups can be a great way for people with diabetes to connect with others and learn more about managing their condition. a long note about diabetic support groups

Chapter 9

Diabetes Education Programs

Diabetes education programs are essential for people living with diabetes to help them better manage their condition and improve their overall health. Diabetes affects millions of people worldwide and is a chronic and complex disease that requires ongoing management.

Diabetes education programs provide people with the tools and resources they need to better understand their condition and make informed decisions about their health.

Diabetes education programs typically include a comprehensive approach to diabetes care and management. They provide information about diabetes and its management, including nutrition, physical activity, and medications.

Education programs also incorporate lifestyle changes such as reducing stress, smoking cessation, and improving sleep. People living with diabetes also learn about their rights, resources, and support systems.

A successful diabetes education program should be tailored to the individual's needs and should be provided by an interdisciplinary team of health professionals. This team should include a pharmacist, dietitian, nurse, mental health professional, and physician.

The program should be tailored to the individual's cultural and socioeconomic background to ensure that the patient is able to apply the information and strategies to their own lives.

Education programs should be ongoing and provide support throughout the patient's journey with diabetes. This includes providing access to resources and support groups, as well as offering follow-up visits.

It is also important to provide ongoing education and coaching so that individuals can keep up with the latest developments in diabetes management.

Diabetes education programs are essential for people living with diabetes. They provide the tools and resources needed to help people better manage their condition, improve their overall health, and lead a healthier life.

Chapter 10

Diabetes-Friendly Recipes

Diabetes-friendly recipes are an excellent way to maintain a healthy diet while managing diabetes. Eating a healthy diet can help keep blood sugar levels in check and reduce the risk of complications associated with diabetes.

Eating a variety of healthy foods can also help people with diabetes feel better, have more energy, and maintain a healthy weight.

When planning meals, people with diabetes should focus on eating a variety of foods, including lean proteins, whole grains, legumes, fruits, vegetables, and healthy fats.

It is important to include a balance of carbohydrates, proteins, and fats in each meal. People with diabetes should also limit their intake of foods that are high in saturated fats, trans fats, sodium, and added sugars.

When eating carbohydrates, it is important to choose complex carbohydrates, such as whole grains, legumes, and starchy vegetables. These foods are broken down slowly, which helps keep blood sugar levels stable.

Eating foods that are high in fiber can also help to slow down digestion, which helps to maintain blood sugar levels.

In addition to choosing the right foods, people with diabetes should also pay attention to portion sizes. It is important to keep portion sizes in check in order to keep blood sugar levels in an acceptable range.

People with diabetes should also spread out their carbohydrate intake throughout the day, as eating too many carbohydrates at once can cause blood sugar levels to rise.

Finally, people with diabetes should be sure to stay hydrated. Drinking plenty of water throughout the day can help to keep blood sugar levels in check. It is also important to avoid sugary drinks, such as soda and juice, as they can cause blood sugar levels to spike.

Eating a healthy diet that is tailored to the needs of people with diabetes can help to keep blood sugar levels stable and reduce the risk of complications associated with diabetes.

With some careful planning and an understanding of which foods are best for managing diabetes, people with diabetes can enjoy a variety of delicious and healthy meals.

Additional resources

1. The American Diabetes Association: This is the leading organization for providing resources and support to individuals living with diabetes. They offer a variety of resources such as health information, recipes, and tips for managing diabetes. They also provide support groups, educational materials, and advocacy efforts.

2. Diabetes.org: This website is an online hub for the latest news, research, and resources related to diabetes. It contains articles, recipes, and a community forum for those living with diabetes. It also offers a library of resources that covers everything from medication to nutrition to lifestyle management.

3. Centers for Disease Control and Prevention (CDC): The CDC provides a wealth of information related to diabetes prevention and management, including statistics, guidelines, and research.They also provide resources to help members of the public understand diabetes, their risk factors, and how to prevent or manage the condition.

4. National Institute of Diabetes and Digestive and Kidney Diseases (NIDDK): The NIDDK is a government agency that provides research and resources related to diabetes. They focus on the

causes, treatments, and prevention of diabetes as well as its complications.

5. Joslin Diabetes Center: This center is a leader in diabetes care and research. They provide comprehensive care and offer educational materials, lifestyle advice, and resources. They also have a variety of research initiatives, clinical trials, and support groups.

6. American Association of Diabetes Educators: This association accredits diabetes educators and provides resources for people with diabetes and those who care for them.

7. Diabetes Research Institute: This organization is dedicated to researching treatments and cures for diabetes.

8. WebMD: This website provides comprehensive information about diabetes, including nutrition, exercise, and medications.

9. Mayo Clinic: This website provides detailed information about diabetes, including diagnosis, treatments, and lifestyle changes.

10. My Diabetes Home: This website is a comprehensive online platform for managing diabetes. It includes tools for tracking blood glucose levels, medications, and meals.

Conclusion

The diabetic cookbook is a valuable resource for anyone looking to improve their health and lifestyle. With its easy-to-follow recipes, it is a great way to start on a journey to better health.

It offers delicious and nutritious recipes that are easy to make, allowing for more time to focus on other aspects of life. Additionally, it provides helpful tips, techniques, and advice for managing diabetes, all of which can be used for a lifetime of healthy eating.

With its comprehensive approach to diabetes, this cookbook is an invaluable resource for those living with the condition. By taking the time to learn what works best for the individual, and by using this cookbook as a guide, one can successfully manage diabetes and lead a healthy and fulfilling life.